BREAKING THE ITCH-SCRATCH CYCLE OF ECZEMA BY BEHAVIOR MODIFICATION

BREAKING THE ITCH-SCRATCH CYCLE OF ECZEMA BY BEHAVIOR MODIFICATION

DOCTOR BEE, M.D.

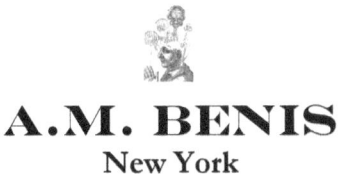

A.M. BENIS
New York

Die Methode ist alles.
(It's all in the method.)
— Carl Ludwig (1816-1895)

CONTENTS

ILLUSTRATIONS

PREFACE

As the reader may have guessed, this little book is the result of a physician's personal experience with a common problem, namely that of dealing with the itch-scratch cycle associated with a chronic skin condition. After years of half-measures — and half-baked measures — I finally concluded that I needed to face the issue before my condition became really serious, and what I lacked was a clear-cut method of dealing with it.

My first "Aha!" moment came when I noticed that the itching, and of course the urge to scratch the guilty area, was greatly diminished when I was driving a car. "Of course," I reasoned. "My brain is processing a lot of information associated with driving, so the itching gets low priority and is virtually ignored!" So, in principle at least, the solution was simple: just overload the brain with stimuli whenever you have an itching episode, and the sensation will be "blocked". The question, of course, was how to do this in a practical manner. Going through the motions of driving a car every time you get an itch might not be the best way!

My next step was a journey backwards in time to my medical school training in the neurosciences. Although every physician who does not specialize in this area quickly forgets most of the material, there is one image in the field of neurology that stays with every medical student forever. This is Wilder Penfield's somewhat whimsical "homunculus" (see the figures in Chapter 3). This "little man" is a grossly distorted representation of the human body, where the sizes of the various body parts are either enlarged or reduced according to how much brain matter is associated with their function. Indeed, it was impossible for me not to remember that sensation and movement of a person's *fingers and hands* are hugely disproportionate in the homunculus. This, then, was the second clue to our puzzle, namely that focusing on the function of one's hands may be the key to blocking the sensation of itching.

It only remained for us to optimize a method of "behavior modification", specifically to break the itch-scratch cycle, and that is the subject of this booklet. The scheme that we devised worked very well for us, but will it work for most people? Will it work for you? Will it be effective in other, sometimes very diffuse skin conditions like psoriasis, or in severe, localized conditions like scrotal lichenificaton?

It is too early to give an answer to the above questions, but on the optimistic side we can see no reason why the method should not work for a wide variety of skin disorders. How effective the technique will be for a given individual may depend on personality factors. Introspective, perfectionistic individuals might have an advantage here. But, a positive outcome is likely more dependent on one's motivation to succeed than on any specific personality trait that one might have.

And so, on this optimistic note we wish you, the reader, "Good luck and Godspeed".

1

Introduction

Our objective is to present an easily followed method to break the *itch-scratch cycle* that often plagues individuals who suffer from various skin disorders, and in particular, eczema. We assume that you have already been diagnosed by a physician, that you are fairly knowledgeable, and that you have already been through all sorts of internet searches and unsuccessful trials of salves, creams, bathing rituals, and whatnot. You quietly smile to yourself, or roll your eyes, when your doctor says, "… and by the way, try not to scratch." Perhaps you have a trouble spot in a particular intimate area that no one else knows about, and you suffer in silence. Perhaps you have been blaming yourself for just not having the "will power" to refrain from scratching. Perhaps the condition is getting worse. Perhaps you are at wits' end.

The method

Our aim is to be clear, brief and concise, without a lot of pontificating or telling you what you already know. Here are the essentials of the method:

- Accepting, starting today, that scratching is no longer an option,

- a technique of blocking sensory inputs so that the sensation of itching is suppressed,

- shifting the focus from the troublesome area of your body to the tips of your fingers and the palms of your hands,

- modifying your behavior with the use of a punishment/reward scheme, and

- attention to nighttime and to matters of daily routine.

Consult your physician

No advice pertaining to a medical problem is appropriate for everyone. Ask your doctor if a trial of our method is appropriate for you. If you are using topical products that are simply not working, this might be a good time to try something different. But do not stop any medications on your own. Talk to your doctor first.

2

The Concepts

The itch-scratch cycle

The itch-scratch cycle involves what system analysts call "positive feedback", which occurs when the result of a process enhances the effect of the original stimulus. A good example is sexual activity. When positive feedback is in control, the system is not in stable equilibrium, and something has got to give.

In the case of the scratch-itch cycle, it is the process of scratching that enhances the original sensation of itching. The ill-desired result is often an area of skin that is sensitive, inflamed, discolored, thickened and excoriated, or as the dermatologists would say "… with a loss of barrier integrity".

But a system where positive feedback is operative is vulnerable. If the "feedback loop" is interrupted, then the system can be restored to equilibrium, and indeed that is our objective. Specifically, in order to break the itch-scratch cycle we shall block the sensation of itching that drives the process of scratching.

Behavioral modification

Human behavior can be rather complicated, with elements of both unconscious and conscious behavior that are often inextricably entwined. In the case of unconscious behavior, it is a matter of "the brain telling you what to do, and you just go ahead and do it." In the case of conscious behavior, the tables are reversed: it is "you who tell the brain what you want done".

Behavioral modification hinges on the fact that we are conscious, cognitive beings who can devise ways to deal with our behavior, especially when it comes to acts that we do by habit. In our method, it is we who *consciously take control* of elements of our behavior that seemed beyond our control.

Punishment and reward

Schemes of behavioral modification can involve both reward and punishment, or as psychologists would say, "positive reinforcement". In our method, we do incorporate punishments, but they are very mild ones, being more in the category of incentives or inconveniences. Nevertheless, we shall call them "punishments" to demonstrate our seriousness of purpose.

Our method does not give out "little rewards" on a day-to-day basis. However, the system is intrinsically self-rewarding. It will be a satisfaction to know that one has a technique on hand for alleviating itching, wherever and whenever it should occur. And what could be more rewarding than an improvement in one's general health?

Infraction and relapse

Our objective is to prevent the occurrence of habitual scratching. If such an undesirable incident does occur, it is termed an "infraction" (the word "failure" seems unduly harsh). If an incident occurs after a long scratch-free period, it is termed a "relapse". In our method, infractions and relapses are subject to punishment.

Early in treatment, we require that for an "infraction" to have occurred, actual scratching must have taken place. Later on, if we even unconsciously *touch* the affected area, this is considered to be an infraction. And, yes, it is subject to punishment.

A common reason for the occurrence of a relatively serious infraction will be when, due to distraction or stress, one unconsciously begins to caress or lightly scratch the troublesome area. This has a high probability of degenerating into a full-blown scratching event because once scratching has started, it will be virtually impossible to interrupt until it has run its full course. For this reason, just the touching of the affected area is considered (later in treatment) as seriously as an actual incident of scratching.

Daily routines

A good part of our daily lives resides in routines, especially our nighttime routines, so this is an important issue that will need to be addressed in any treatment plan.

Starting "cold turkey"

Our method does not require any training or habituation. You can begin without delay.

If not now, then when?

Even a journey of a thousand miles begins with a single step. Let's get started.

3

Block the itch!

Stimulus and response

Much of what one reads about the itch-scratch cycle is rather muddled, as if itching and scratching were equal entities on the opposite sides of a coin. This is not true. Itching is a *sensation*, while scratching is a *response* to the sensation, driving the "feedback loop" that enhances the original sensation and threatens to destroy the integrity of the system.

There are two basic ways that the itch-scratch cycle can be interrupted.

One could try in a brute force way, by sheer will power, resolve to stop scratching. Or you could tie your arms behind your back, or bundle your hands, hoping that if you prevent yourself from scratching, the cycle will be interrupted. You have high hopes that the troublesome area will begin to heal, and the itching sensation will gradually resolve itself. Maybe you have already tried something like this.

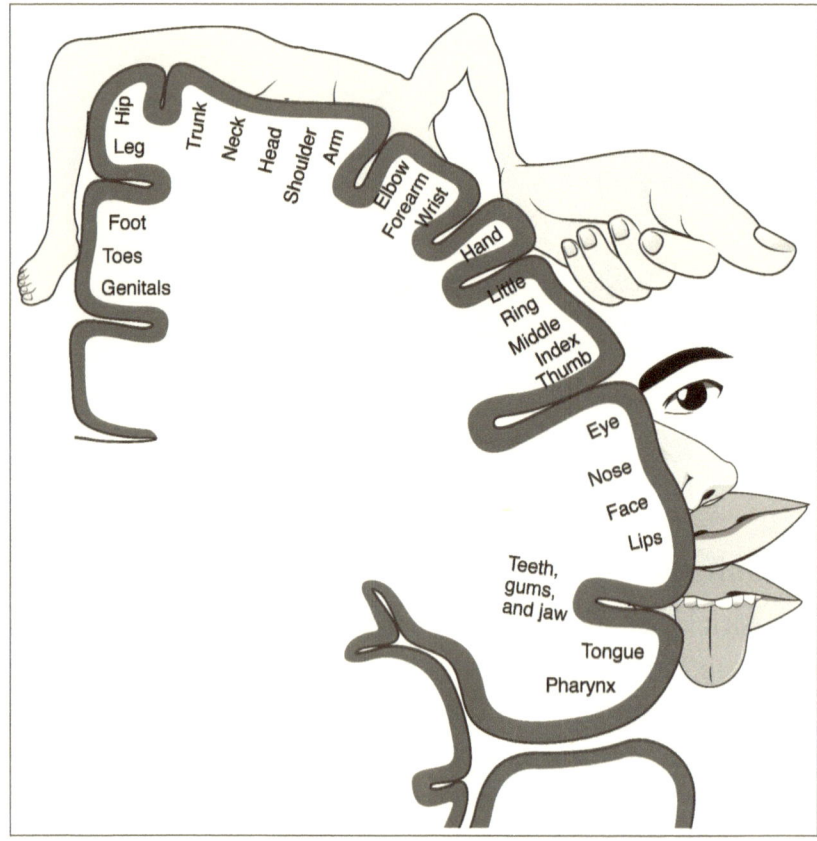

Fig. 1. Penfield's map, showing the association of parts of the body with the areas of the brain where sensation is processed. The bold, dark outline represents the exterior of the cerebral cortex. Note the large representation of the hands and face. [*Wikipedia Commons*]

The second way to interrupt the cycle, and the one that we shall use, involves *blocking the sensation of itching,* rather than trying to rein in the runaway horse of scratching.

The brain is a computer

Like your personal computer, the brain is pretty good at multitasking. But it has limits. Our premise is that if we explore the limits of the brain in the processing of sensory inputs, of which itching is one, then we can come up with a scheme where itching is given low priority, or essentially blocked.

Our vision of the brain being "too busy" to process the sensory input of itching while we are driving a car is no doubt a simplistic one. One day neuroscientists will explain what is occurring in formal terms, using such terms as "neurotransmitters" and "inhibitory synapses". However, for our purposes we will be content, at present, to accept the simple explanation.

Penfield's homunculus

The homunculus, the little model of a man derived from the neurosurgical experiments of Wilder Penfield, is shown in Figures 1 and 2. As we mentioned in the Preface, the homunculus has physical features that are proportioned according to the amount of brain tissue is allotted to their function. My, my, what big hands he has!

What you may have not realized immediately is that the homunculus depicted in Figure 2 is actually the very image of… *you.* That's right, it is a faithful picture of you, and it is you who has hands that are very large, very sensitive and very sensuous. We shall put them to good use.

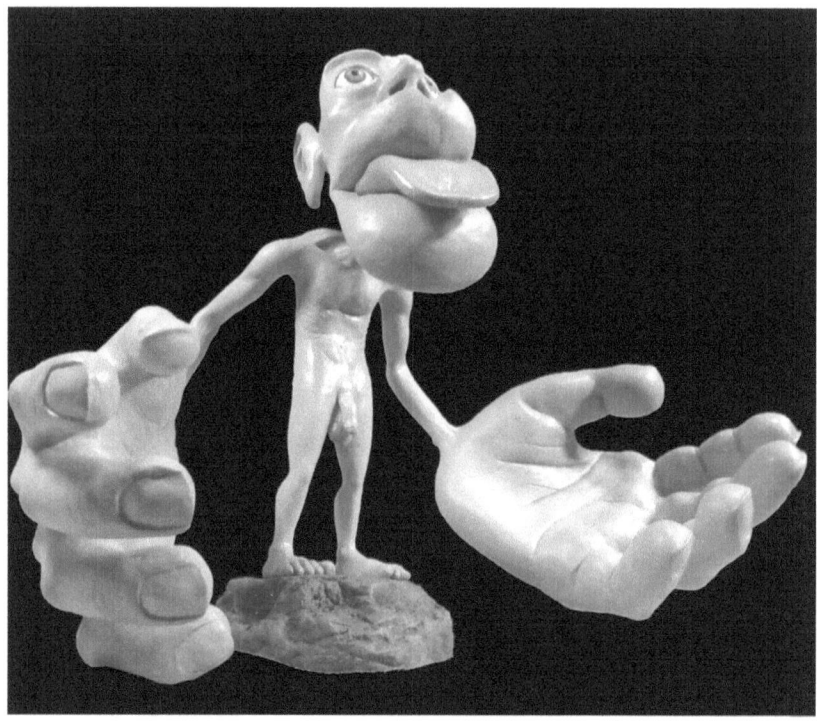

Fig. 2. The "sensory homunculus", a physical model of a human based on Figure 1, where the size of body parts are proportional to corresponding areas of the brain where sensation is processed. Note the especially large hands. [*Wikipedia Commons*]

Hand stimulation

Here is how it works.

When you have the sensation of itching in your troublesome area, normally you would instinctively touch the area, maybe with an intent to mildly scratch or maybe (trying to fool yourself) just with an intent to caress the itch into submission.

However, that is not what you are going to do any longer. Instead, you will bring your hands together and mutually stimulate them. Using your fingertips, you will tickle, caress or scratch, using one hand to stimulate the other, usually for time no longer than 30 seconds. For maximum stimulation, one can firmly scratch the palms of both hands. You will pleasingly note that the itching sensation was blocked… and you wonder "… for how long?"

Well, nobody knows for how long the itching will subside, but it was a rather benign procedure, so we shall repeat it as often as necessary.

Note that we are trying to interrupt the itch-scratch cycle as it pertains to a particular problematic area of the body. We do not mean to suggest that the technique should be used for benign tickles and itches in other parts of the body.

The hand stimulation technique has a threefold function:

1. It blocks the sensation of itching.

2. It physically redirects the focus from the problem area of your body to your large, lovely and sensuous hands.

3. It puts you in the driver's seat. You are in control, rather than just being a blind, obedient servant of your brain. Scratching the palms of your hands sends a subtle message to your brain. It is "Yes, I am scratching. But I am scratching in the time and location of my own choosing!"

The technique

If you are alone, it is very easy. You can use the fingertips of one hand to tickle, caress or scratch the opposite hand. There are a thousand ways of doing this, and you can decide what is best for you. You can even extend the stimulation to your wrists and lower forearms.

If you are not alone, clasp both hands together with thumbs interlocked and the fingers not interlaced. You will note that the thumb of one hand lies in the palm of the other, while the index finger of the other hand similarly lies in the palm of its opposite. This is a perfect position for tickling or scratching the palms of both hands. The stimulation can be very effective, and no one else present will have the slightest idea of what you are doing, wherever you may be.

If you do not have both hands free and cannot bring them together, you can still curl the fingers of each hand to stimulate the palms.

Wow, it works!

The hand stimulation technique is just a tool. We still need to incorporate it in a workable method for breaking the itch-scratch cycle. And this is the subject of the next chapter.

4

Modify Your Behavior

Three steps to success

In order to succeed in an endeavor, it helps to have the right tool, but that is not enough. We need a method by which we can optimize its use and evaluate its efficacy.

As the first step in the treatment plan you agree to acknowledge that you are embarking on a new approach, with a heightened awareness of the various issues associated with the itch-scratch cycle. In very stark terms, you acknowledge, "cold turkey" style, that *scratching is no longer an option.*

The second step is to *begin using the hand stimulation technique*, to get to know how it works best for you.

The third step is to optimize the use of the hand stimulation technique so that, as rapidly as possible, we reach our goal of a healed troublesome area of the body, with the itch-scratch problem relegated to obscurity, or at least to the level of a minor problem. To achieve this, we shall use an aspect of *behavioral modification* known as punishment.

Do not be alarmed by the word "punishment". No electric shocks will be administered. If anyone asks, tell them that our method sometimes uses "mild redirection to suppress unwanted behaviorisms".

Evaluate infractions and relapses

We define an *infraction* as an incident where scratching occurs, whether it is started consciously or unconsciously. As we mentioned earlier, as time goes on and healing of the affected area improves, you should be stricter with yourself and treat any unconscious touching of the area as an infraction.

Infractions can be of various severity, which we grade on a scale of 1+ to 4+. A 1+ incident would correspond to touching the area or starting to scratch, while a 4+ incident would be a full-blown relapse to scratching that runs its course. Incidents getting a 2+ or 3+ rating would be somewhere in between.

Because of the rather complicated lives that most of us lead, infractions and relapses are to be expected. They should not be treated as "failures" but simply as (ho-hum) expected episodes in any serious treatment program.

Dealing with infractions

The best way to deal with infractions and relapses will depend on the individual, and you will need to decide what is best for you. The following threefold "punishment" scheme worked well for us, but you may wish to modify it. Here are the three categories:

1. An immediate response to an infraction

2. Mandatory bathroom care

3. Keeping a log of infractions

Immediate response to an infraction — Our method of dealing with infractions is unusual in that it incorporates the method of stimulus suppression (the hand stimulation technique) into the punishment scheme.

Here is how it works. If an infraction occurs, such as your unconsciously starting to scratch while reading a newspaper, the punishment is *doing the hand stimulation technique for 30 seconds while holding your hands above your head.*

This classifies as a "punishment" because it forces you to interrupt what you are doing, and it forces you into a somewhat awkward physical position that would be embarrassing if someone were to observe you. However, the scheme also acts as a positive reinforcement in the three ways mentioned earlier: 1) it acts to suppress the itching stimulus, which was of course the culprit of the whole affair, 2) it redirects the focus from the troublesome area to your hands, and 3) it reemphasizes that you are in control by your voluntary actions.

The above hand stimulation response would be appropriate if you were alone. If you are not alone, then you have two options. First, you could substitute the clasped hands technique (p. 12) without raising your hands above your head, or second, you could postpone the 30 second punishment until a later time.

Mandatory bathroom care — In the event of a full-blown (4+) relapse, the punishment is a repeat of your usual bathroom ritual that you do every day in dealing with your condition. This could be something like lathering the affected area with a "body wash", waiting 5 minutes, and then taking a shower. This classifies as a "punishment" because you are forced to interrupt your routine to do it (as soon as you are able), but it also has the positive aspect of freshly "resetting" the condition of your skin, so that you are ready to continue with renewed determination.

Keeping a log of infractions — If you are the type of person who hates to keep meticulous records, then it will, indeed, be a punishment to keep a log of infractions as they occur. But there can be a positive aspect to keeping such a log, especially later on when one looks back with nostalgia at the old frequent entries and admires how far one has progressed.

In the Appendix we give an outline of what a log could look like, but you may wish to start your own separate log book. The "score" column could be a number from 1 to 10 that describes how well you judge your progress to date, irrespective of the infraction or relapse that occurred that particular day.

Keeping the wolf at bay

The above responses focus on how we should treat specific instances as they haphazardly occur on difficult days. However, we can do much in the way of how we manage our *daily routines* to ensure that the ogre of the itch-scratch cycle does not show his face again… and that is the subject of the next chapter.

5

Daily Routines

Bathroom routine

By bathroom routine we mean the ritual that you do every day in dealing with your condition. It may be a rather complicated, time-consuming affair, employing a variety of topical applications. As your condition improves, you may suspect that maybe you don't need this or that procedure anymore and that you could greatly simply your bathroom ritual. This may turn out to be true, but consult with your doctor first.

Nighttime routine

Nighttime is always problematic for those who suffer from dermatologic conditions, and for good reason. At night, the areas of the brain devoted to sensory and motor activity (feeling and movement) do not have much else to do, other than to process all those itchy sensations coming from that troublesome, inflamed area of your body.

Happily, the hand stimulation technique can be used at night, as well. If you are awakened at night with an itching sensation, you can use the "separate hands" technique in which you curl the fingers of each hand to stimulate the palms for a few seconds (see p. 12). This may be enough to block the itch and send you back to sleep. Early in treatment one should not expect to eliminate all episodes of nighttime scratching but rather to reduce their frequency. If episodes of untoward scratching do occur during a particular night, one should consider that to be an infraction and perform a 30-second period of hand stimulation "punishment" (p. 15) on arising in the morning.

If your problem area is on the thighs, between the legs or on the midriff, then try sleeping on your side with a large, soft pillow wedged very firmly between your legs. This has the effect of protecting the area from unconscious scratching, and the tight fit also tends to suppress the "tickling" aspect that occurs at the onset of many episodes of itching.

Preemptive hand stimulation

Several times a day, when nothing much is going on, scratch the palms of your hands for a few seconds. The purpose of this is to remind your brain that you are in control here and that you are ready for anything that it might throw at you... in the category of itching.

Closing note

It is remarkable that the use of hand stimulation to suppress itching is not common knowledge. A literature search produces no citations. Perhaps the technique was known to the ancients but has been lost to the passage of time.

6

Summary

- Consult your physician to verify that our treatment plan of behavior modification is appropriate for you.

- In the itch-scratch cycle, itching is a sensation, while scratching is a response with positive feedback.

- We describe a technique of hand stimulation that can be used to block the sensation of itching.

- The hand stimulation technique has a threefold function: it blocks the itching, it shifts the focus from the area of itching to the hands, and it reminds you that you are in control.

- If you decide to try this method, accept that you need to devise a specific plan or protocol that is appropriate for you.

- Step 1: Accept that scratching is no longer an option.

- Step 2: Learn and practice the hand stimulation technique.

- Step 3: Optimize the technique of hand stimulation by using a method of behavior modification. Our method involves "positive reinforcement" that includes mild "punishments" for infractions and relapses.

- Expect that infractions and relapses will occur. Accept that they are routinely anticipated and dealt with in the treatment plan.

- Pay attention to daily routines. Maintain a heightened awareness that you are undergoing a treatment plan of behavioral modification. Practice "preemptive hand stimulation" several times a day, even on days when you have no symptoms of itching.

- And finally… reward yourself when you attain a scratch-free period of six months duration. Splurge. Bring out the champagne! You do not need the permission of your brain. Just go ahead and do it.

APPENDIX
Personal log

<u>date</u>	<u>outcome</u>	<u>score</u>

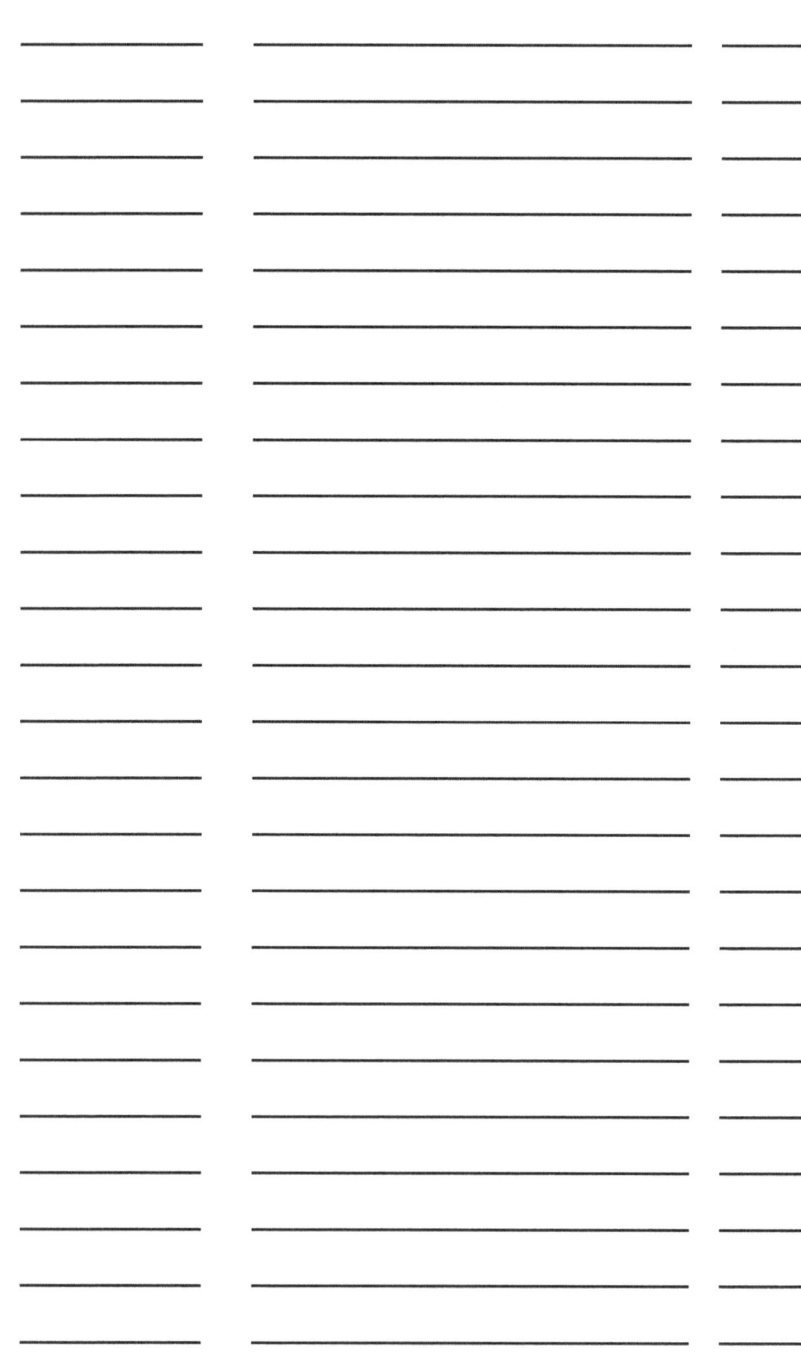

GLOSSARY

behavior modification   A treatment approach that replaces undesirable modes of behavior with more desirable ones, with the use of learning techniques, rewards and punishments. Also called *cognitive behavioral therapy.*

cerebral cortex   The outer layer of the two hemispheres of the brain.

cognition   The acts of thinking, feeling, knowing, reasoning and learning, including both awareness and judgment.

feedback, positive   When the output of a system enhances the effect of the original stimulus.

hand stimulation technique   In the present method, the manual self-stimulation of the hands in order to block the stimulus of itching.

homunculus   Refers to the model of the human body according to the data of W. Penfield, where the various body parts are distorted in proportion to the amount of cerebral cortex devoted to their functions.

infraction   In the present method, an incident of touching or scratching of the affected area during treatment.

itch-scratch cycle   In the itch-scratch cycle itching is a sensation, while scratching is a response with positive feedback.

itching   An irritating sensation caused by sensory receptors in the skin and subject to temporary relief by stimulation of the affected area by rubbing or scratching.

motor   Refers to parts of the nervous system that control movement.

Penfield, Wilder (1891-1976)   American-Canadian neurosurgeon who developed the concept of the cortical homunculus.

preemptive stimulation   In the present method, use of the hand stimulation technique, whenever one chooses, during times when there is no bothersome itching.

reinforcement   Establishing a pattern of behavior, especially by reward or punishment.

relapse   A recurrence of an incident of scratching after a prolonged period of scratch-free behavior.

sensation   The body's detection of an internal or external stimulus.

sensory   Pertaining to the senses. The five classical senses are sight, smell, hearing, taste, and touch, but there are many others. Itching is most related to touch.

stimulus   A cause of a physiological response. §

SOURCES OF ILLUSTRATIONS

Figure 1. OpenStax College. From Anatomy and Physiology, via *Wikipedia Commons.* Connexions web site. http://cnx.org/content/col11496/1.6/.

Figure 2. By Mpj29. CC BY-SA 4.0, via *Wikipedia Commons.* http://creativecommons.org/licenses/by-sa/4.0.

ABOUT THE AUTHOR

Dr. Bee (pseudonym) is a retired physician and biomedical researcher. He served for many years as research associate professor and director of cardiac intensive care at a major medical center in New York City.